THE ROCKY ROAD TO PEACE AND PURPOSE

(NEW EDITION)

Sylvia Bryden-Stock

Author's Tranquility Press
Marietta, Georgia

Sylvia Bryden-Stock/Author's Tranquility Press
2706 Station Club Drive SW
Marietta, GA 30060
www.authorstranquilitypress.com

Ordering Information:
Quantity sales. Special discounts are available on quantity purchases by corporations, associations, and others. For details, contact the "Special Sales Department" at the address above.

THE ROCKY ROAD TO PEACE AND PURPOSE/ Sylvia Bryden-Stock
Paperback: 978-1-957208-93-0
eBook: 978-1-957208-94-7

To Live in the Moment and Be at Peace
is
The Very Best Life Goal to Work At

CONTENTS

FOREWORD

Although well studied and understood, dementia is still an extremely challenging situation for the person, carer, and everyone else around.

I have known Sylvia for many years since Brian was in our care for almost six years. She was also a volunteer at the home; educating our staff and constantly offering an unlimited source of support for each of our relatives who were struggling with their loved one's diagnosis of dementia and admittance to a Care Home.

For us, Sylvia is a person who is always there to educate carers and family members to better cope with the psychological and emotional challenges of living with dementia. Having witnessed Brian living with Young Onset Alzheimer's Disease and facing the emotions of being a Carer in her own life.

Princess Christian Care Centre is a home where many residents live with dementia, and for us, it was a blessing that Sylvia was offering this support to the families and Carers of residents in our Care Home.

In her previous book, 'The rocky road of Naughty Neurons' Sylvia helped her readers to identify the common challenges of a dementia diagnosis and the life there after, from a carer's perspective. Her suggestions on dealing with the situation are helpful for anyone who is a carer or living with the condition.

I believe that the immense positivity Sylvia shares through this new book; 'The rocky road to Peace and Purpose' will help the readers, as a carer and a life companion, to find themselves in a better mind-set dealing with the late stages of dementia particularly when it reaches the stages of bereavement and grief.

I wish Sylvia all the very best with this new book and would like to thank her for her work which I hope will be useful to millions of carers in overcoming the challenges of living with dementia.

With love,

Mario Taherian
registered Manager rGN, MSC
Princess Christian Care Centre
Woking

INTRODUCTION

It's a coolish but sunny day here at Rye Harbour Park Homes Holiday Park. The Platinum Grade caravan I am staying in is "heaven sent", with full central heating and double glazing, en-suite in the main bedroom plus a beautifully furnished kitchen with integrated appliances and top of the range hob and double oven. Literally home from home and offered at a bargain rate!

The site is adjacent to a beautiful nature reserve which affords a sense of peace, with walks out to the Rye Estuary and harbour entrance. I recall a previous stay here with my husband during the turmoil we went through prior to getting married (see The Rocky Road of Naughty Neurons), when he had some challenges, but mental capacity was not compromised. We had come to have a chill-out and de-stress after being told a third time, that, due to a caveat being placed on our wedding, more evidence was needed.

This time I am here on my own to "tap into God's peace and create". You see, Brian went home to heaven recently – as I believe there is a better place for us when we leave our physical body – and I am taking a few days out to begin the journey of adapting to a new phase of my life that also has a great purpose to it.

The journey with my husband, although painful to watch, has been an amazing teacher, plus, generated a service to humanity, a ministry dedicated to helping

Carers deal with those turbulent emotions that are part of watching someone you love travel the cruel journey of Alzheimer's Disease or other form of Dementia (https://dementia-whisperer.com).

Get ready to share my journey through the late stages of Young Onset Alzheimer's Disease; how I grew emotionally stronger and adapted to major change and finally gave my husband permission to step out of his physical body that, indeed, had not served him well for a number of years.

Once again you will learn how I dealt with circumstances and the ability to find inner peace in times of deep distress, stepping from being a victim to walking in victory.

During the late stages, it is like stepping on to an even greater roller coaster of emotions. However, if you have been able to, in any way, conquer the previous ones, the basic strategy will help with the pending emotional roller coaster.

Just think for a moment – Have you dealt with other life traumas and got through? Did fear initially step in saying "I can't do this!" Or "How can I get through this?"

This journey is another life experience that will at times have a sense of being in the middle of the ocean with no land in sight. A way to deal with the storm has to be sought, and the ability to find those deep down calm waters of Inner Peace.

Sometimes it can seem like you deal with one storm, sail into those Inner calm Waters of Peace, when yet another storm situation arises! Oh My! Got to get riding this one now and tap into the Inner Peace yet again!

This is what you will see illustrated as I share the final part of my husband's Alzheimer's journey and the strategies I created to ongoing Peace and begin turning "Pain into Purpose"

PART 1

Till Transition Time Comes

<u>CHAPTER 1</u>

Transitioning to New Experiences

I was visiting my husband at Princess Christian Care Home for lunch as usual on a Friday. The Care Home Manager saw me arriving and asked how long I was staying as he wanted to have a chat with me.

Do you remember school days or workdays when you were asked to "have a chat"? Isn't it interesting how instinctively you expect the absolute worst? Definitely in trouble over something!

Well, my immediate inner response was a similar feeling, especially as Brian was now in the latter stages of his Young Onset Alzheimer's Disease journey. Choosing not to dwell on it, I went into his unit and fed him, enjoyed my own lunch of salmon and vegetables, and after spending some time with him went to see the Care Home Manager. We have a great rapport and having been in the same position as him some years ago, I respected the fact that he might have some sensitive issues to discuss.

After a brief, typical chat we would usually have, he then put to me a recommendation for my husband -

"Sylvia, I have had a meeting with Brian's unit Head Nurse and Deputy Manager and we feel that Brian is a full nursing care resident and it would be better for him to be upstairs in the Nursing Wing" This had been put to me back in February of 2018 and we created a compromise whereby Brian would be resident in the nursing wing and come down to his old unit for most of the day – he was used to the staff and their voices. Also, this had been his place of residence since admission in November of 2014. However, this time, I agreed to have my husband to stay in the nursing unit full time for his nursing needs to be suitably met. They had also provided him with a "banana chair" that was both comfortable and safe for him to be in during the day. The chair was also able to be wheeled around facilitating the ability to take him down to his old unit for a time if it was feasible.

He settled into his new surroundings and gradually established a rapport with all the staff through voice recognition as his Posterior Cortex Atrophy fully prevented visual acuity. This was why I negotiated a compromise routine on his initial move to the nursing wing so that he could visit old familiar voices and senses during part of the day.

Alzheimer's patients can sense change, and in my husband's case the visual issues would affect how he responded to new people and surroundings. I was relieved when my compromise suggestion was put in place.

A positive in his move was the lovely light and spacious room overlooking the care park and meadowland which, although not able to be seen by Brian, would facilitate great space for future visiting by myself and family and friends, especially when he would be fully bed bound.

Now facing a new challenge of adjustment and acceptance, I had to deal with a new set of emotions associated with facing ongoing deterioration with his Alzheimer's Disease along with watching him go through challenges of compliance around interactions needed with people and new sounds. A sense of comfort came from the compromise situation until – the day I witnessed his "naughty neutrons" behaviour and another challenge whilst downstairs in his more familiar surroundings.

By now he was having grade one thickening to his drinks as there was a typical swallowing reflex issue beginning to develop with him. This could cause coughing fits when drinks were being administered as well as during meals.

As per usual I joined him for lunch one day and fed him the carefully finely chopped and mashed lunch. During his first course he began to cough and was almost choking with colour changes. The nurse and Carers dealt with the situation and a dietary and fluid review was urgently requested.

It can be very upsetting to witness circumstances that indicate signs of deterioration in your loved one's condition with a "fear of change" and acceptance of new manifestations. Adjustment to change has already taken place and emotional responses plateaued and then a new challenge arises within the emotional roller coaster ride.

I have always believed that we have a choice regarding how we deal with life's challenges. You see, life does throw up challenges in many aspects of day to day living. It's not what is happening, it is our response to what is happening that is most important.

In my situation on that day of seeing a new manifestation with my husband, I decided to override fear with ongoing belief in the amazing care he was receiving along with any blessings to be found in amongst the transition of disease manifestation and necessary care management adjustments.

Do you actively look for even the smallest of blessings in life? Here are a few blessings I decided to focus on at this time of yet another hurdle to face –

- Brian still knew who I was and could, in his way, let me know his love for me in amongst manifesting anger and frustration.

- The staff were giving heart centered care and had genuine concern for both Brian and myself.

- I was kept informed of any changes and minor issues observed e.g developing a boil on his buttocks that required antibiotic treatment.

Seeking out and observing blessings in life every day, brings a sense of inner peace and joy which helps you cope during those difficult times. It does take dedicated daily effort but the rewards on the emotional roller coaster ride are worth it.

The overall blessing for me was that Brian was being cared for in a place that had extremely high standards of care, continually monitoring and implementing positive improvements. I could "sleep at night" knowing that he was in safe and loving-care by all. By now the relationship I had with all the staff from Manager down to cleaning and laundry and kitchen, was one of being part of a family.

Knowing this, I made a conscious decision to embrace change over which I had no control except my response.

I did go through quite an inner adjustment at this time and felt a sense of loss initially over my own need to learn to trust the new staff and the changing routine which was in the very best interest of my husband's ongoing nursing care.

I recall the day when he was down in his previous unit for part of the day and we would have lunch together – I fed him – and spend time together afterwards. After lunch I witnessed Brian's "naughty neurons" kicking in! There were shouting outbursts and major fidgeting in his banana chair. I called a carer and said I would take him back to the nursing wing. I know in my heart that this was goodbye to any further day time visits. The carer kindly said to me "Sylvia, he is like this most days and disturbs the other residents".

It was now time for his full, settling into the nursing unit, and for staff and myself to be prepared for the adjustment behaviour as he got used to new sounds etc. in his new "home".

For me, I would deal with my own emotions and re-affirm to myself that ultimately this was Brian's journey, and my role was to support him through the disease progression. I could not take on board his response to change. I would pray for peace angels to be sent to him and stay with him 24 hours a day. You see, staff agreed with me that deep down he had a sense of awareness that things were not right. The best thing I could do was love him and remind him of great times together.

On this journey we have to learn how to love in spite of what is happening and keep in mind the knowledge that they just might have that sense of awareness from time to time.

CHAPTER 2

Creating Trust and Friendship

So, here we are, about to start what would be the final part of my husband's Alzheimer's journey. No more frequent visits to his old unit, but an opportunity to become part of another Princess Christian Care Home family. Also, opportunity to build trust in the ability to give high standard, quality care.

The morning and nighttime routine were already established, and daytime was spent in the upstairs lounge in his banana chair. I visited regularly and assisted him with his lunch. This would be a meal presented in a way that supported his swallowing challenges, along with fluids offered slowly to facilitate safe swallowing an minimise the risk of a coughing / choking session.

Very quickly there developed a mutual trust and friendship between myself and the staff, as they realised that I was focused more on a team approach and co-operation towards Brian's care. This approach to his care enabled me to have full involvement in any discussions around decisions of necessary changes for his benefit overall during the final phase of his care needs.

How much do you trust people in your life generally? I ask this question because certain life character traits that have become seated in your subconscious mind will spill over to your role as a carer and create an associated attitude towards the care being received by your loved one. Trust and openness lead to a journey of greater inner calm. Throughout times in my life, I had been "too trusting" to the point of "walk-over". However, through bitter experience I developed a balanced approach to dealing with life which became a great asset in the current circumstances. I will admit to having to allow my husband's care needs to take place from a point of view that the staff were trained to the highest standard and followed the Managers great example of heart centred care.

As the days and weeks went by, a great relationship developed with the unit team, and I could see how they grew to love Brain – how he was able to laugh with them and be happy apart from any of the necessary intervention times!

By now his communicating skills had dramatically deteriorated, but, on occasions, he would actually be able to say "thank you" after staff had fed him and given him fluids. I watched him as he gradually built trust and affection for the staff which had a big part to play in my own trust in their care. It was very evident that they really did love the work they were doing and gave of their best with kindness and patience.

To maintain this level of care for a twelve-hour shift is amazing to me, as someone who has worked in the nursing and care sectors for many years. Those who work in the

Alzheimer's and Dementia's arena are gifted and certainly at Princess Christian Care Home, I can only give them the highest praise for always having a smile and understanding the residents trigger points as they carry out personalised care.

As time progressed in the early days of his time in the nursing unit, the staff were noticing that Brian was becoming more restless in his special chair and crying out after a couple of hours – usually after lunch. Observation showed that he could be in pain or discomfort and paracetamol was prescribed for him which helped for a short time. After discussion between staff and myself a decision was made to have hm stay in bed all day on alternate days and monitor the outcomes with his behavioural traits.

Yes, it was a distressing time for me to watch the man I loved beginning to deteriorate more, yet I was still blessed to have him know me when I visited, wanting a hug and a kiss – except, when like any of us, he was having a "bad day" and was very grumpy!

One day, after we had completed the lunchtime routine, I observed him expressing gross discomfort and suggested he go back to bed. Once in bed and paracetamol administered, he calmed down and went off to sleep.

Knowing how staff are trained to co-operate with relatives whenever and wherever possible, I felt that I could talk with them about his day-to-day routine. Understandably it is best for residents to be encouraged to get dressed and go to the lounge for a change of position and socialisation, plus relatives like to see their loved one up and dressed.

Hereby hangs a question – Is this because it helps with their own emotional response to their loved one's journey?

No matter what changes in routine we're becoming necessary with my husband, I was determined to make decisions that benefited him overall. This generated my suggesting that I was happy for Brian to have 24/7 care in bed if it meant he was comfortable and free of pain. This was an emotional challenge for me, and yes, I released my own pain of watching deterioration in his condition with tears at home but coupled with a sense of inner peace that he would be in less discomfort if he was cared for in bed. I discussed this with the staff, and they agreed that Brian would from now on be cared for in his room in bed.

Now, I had to trust that he would have regular interaction during the day and not be left unattended for long periods as he still had a way of responding to voices and in some way interacting with staff. You see, he had always been a people person and loved company. Having his own Barn Dance band gave great opportunity for the gregarious, fun-loving nature to shine!

My trust was honoured by all sectors of staff greeting me on my visits with how they had been in to see Brian and talked with him along with playing music for him. They also left the Television on for background company.

After around three months of my husband moving to the nursing wing, I was adjusting to the change in his care requirements and trust in the staff had grown in their ability to give "five star" care. They also now considered me to be "a part of the family". I would have fun banter with them and give a listening ear to their own ups and downs on occasions. Word had reached them about "Sylvia's listening ear!". They also showed care and concern for my welfare as well. I assured them that my trust in a greater power helped with generating an inner peace and "being in the moment" with life as much as possible. (I am still perfecting it daily!).

It was in the month of October 2018 that I decided to have a seven night break away and went off to Tunisia to relax and recoup. I ensured that the unit had all details of where I was and key contacts back home. So, knowing that my man was in an amazing place offering superb care plus re-assurance from the staff that they would look after him well. I set off on my travels. Of course, I thought about him and my "family" on the unit but was able to chill out and regain energy to continue on our journey together on my return.

I was not only journeying with Brian, but I was also, through my learnings, creating emotional support tools to help other Carers (https://dementia-whisperer.com).

Because I had grown to trust in the care, acknowledged that it was primarily Brian's journey that I was supporting, the choice to take a break was made without bucket loads of guilt!

He was never a man to stifle me or needy of my presence. As well as his time clock being totally messed up at this stage of his condition, I was able to take a break minus my "way back" guilt trip I used to live with.

When we embrace objective trust in life situations, the owner of guilt fades away. On this pathway it is SO important to trust in ourselves that we are doing our very best with the knowledge and life skills we have, and that we can seek our help where needed. Also, we can stand firm in our ability to challenge where we need to in a way that best serves the situation. The more we expect the best good will come to us. Sometimes on this particular road one is travelling a good old-fashioned prayer can help followed by believing everything – yes everything – has a purpose in it somewhere.

CHAPTER 3

Rising Above – Not Giving In!

One thing this Alzheimer's journey teaches us – it certainly taught me – is to be as ready as you can for any challenge that arises along the way; face it head on whist knowing it has the best interest of your loved one at heart.

In the early stages of my husband's diagnosis, the Aricept medication manifested one of its side effects known as Bradycardia. In lay terms the heart rate drops to around 50 or below and you have a fainting episode. To counter this and have Brian on the high dosage of Aricept a pacemaker was inserted with his approval – he still had sufficient mental capacity to make this decision with the consultant. The procedure went well and then follow up checks were put in place for annual battery review and to assess its functioning.

He was now on a nine months to one year check- up. The overall time in the hospital could be anything up to two hours as return transport had to be arranged by an ambulance crew. Now bed bound with his nursing care, potential for extra agitation plus sitting in a standard wheelchair for a long period of time was out of the question. I discussed with the unit head nurse how his September check- up could be best organised. Could he go as a stretcher case? What would that imply in regard to the logistics? It was agreed with the nurse that I would call the cardiology department and alert them to my husband's current situation. My nursing hat went on "There must be a way that a Domiciliary visit can take place!" I thought to myself as I prepared to call cardiology. "After all, the equipment is like a standard electrocardiograph machine with added software which should not present a problem. There must be others who require a Domiciliary visit for their pacemaker check. (This was before remote checking ones had hit the local marketplace).

I phoned the clinic and explained our situation – putting on my nursing background hat again! – and asked about the possibility of someone coming to the Care Home to carry out a pacemaker check. The response was "interesting"! "He has to come to the clinic!" I was curtly told. "There's no way my husband can travel in a wheelchair now and sit for long periods" I explained "He is totally bed bound in Princess Christian Care Home Nursing wing, and in the latter stages of Alzheimer's". The continued response was that no Domiciliary visits could take place and that he HAD to go to the hospital! I could not help but think of other people who would be challenged to get to the clinic. This made me decide, with the support of the Care Home, to write to the head of the cardiology clinic with a copy to the hospital's Chief Executive so that something could be done about the challenge we and others would be facing. The response was to accept my husband as a stretcher case.

The day dawned and Brian had an extra early routine involving getting him fully dressed with a coat and shoes but sitting in bed. I arrived soon after 9am to wait with him for the ambulance. At 9.30am, two cheerful, full of fun ambulance crew arrived. They were wonderful with Brian, fully understanding our dilemma. One of them was really on the ball after hearing of our experience so far. It was decided to get my man in the ambulance and make a call to the hospital to ensure they were expecting him on a stretcher and would meet him on arrival. They did this as with other patients the transport procedure had failed, and patients turned away at the door!

So Brian is transferred to the stretcher and taken down in the lift and out into the ambulance. I was to follow them and meet at the hospital.

What happened next really put to the test my calm peaceable nature. One of the crew re-appeared and greeted me with "MRS. Stock, I am SO SORRY but, when I called the hospital, they were not prepared for Brian's APPOINTMENT, so it has been aborted and a new one has to be made. "We will bring him back for you now." They showed genuine compassion regarding the whole scenario.

Brian was comfortably re-settled in bed and given a drink while I went to chat with the head nurse about the best action to follow with what had taken place. I said that I was happy to write once more to the hospital expressing my dismay at a system that clearly was not working. A constructive complaint went off in the post and I received an apology from head of Cardiology with a new appointment for January 2019.

All went relatively smoothly with this one, except to say that there is more to tell around the "pacemaker check" saga!! At this appointment, in a unit that could accommodate stretchers, two lovely young ladies appeared after about a one hour wait – here it comes! – with what was a Domiciliary pacemaker checking equipment housed in a lovely purple zip fastening case! I commented politely about this and was told that in larger hospitals staff would be sent out to carry out home visits. They were very empathetic and requested that I write in again and push for changes as they were stretched to the limit plus having to do "on call" work at night.

I did write in as they requested, but soon after, things changed with further appointments not necessary. I just hope that my letter helped with procedure and staffing reviews.

Why do I share this experience? Because I believe that it is important that we bring things to the attention of the Healthcare System, to help them re-consider protocol for the future. Give praise for what is good while constructively bringing to the attention of decision makers things that will not just impact on your own situation but others in similar situations. Complaining and moaning about things without being objective gets one nowhere in life. One thing I always respected about Princess Christian Care Home was their positive approach to "complaints". To them it is opportunity to reflect and consider whether any changes need to be made. I have witnessed this firsthand with my husband's care during the latter stages of his journey.

As he required more intensive care and intervention, his initial morning personal care was carried out by the night staff with a check due no later than 10.30am by the day staff. A combination of very restless behaviour along with kidneys that functioned amazingly, frequent continence care and re-positioning was essential. He had a wonderful habit of somehow disappearing under his V shaped pillow with the sheet wrapped round his head plus feet dangling over the padded cot side and one arm trapped between the mattress and padded cot side. Creativity with extra pillows to keep him in a safe position did not solve the issue! I recall arriving at around midday as per usual to assist with his lunch on two consecutive days and it was obvious that the usual high standard of care plus am check had not been carried out.

I spoke with the nurse in charge and expressed my surprise at what I had witnessed, when their care was at a very high standard. To my delight, this was immediately taken care of, and "plan" put in place which prevented future episodes occurring. For my part I made sure that I thanked the Carers for how good they made Brian look and how much I appreciated the challenge it was for them to work with his resistance when carrying out his care needs. Sometimes he would have had his full care input with added intervention by the morning staff, but when I arrived would require his pad changed again plus re-positioning for lunch – we hoped he maintained it throughout! What was great was that regardless of lunch serving having begun, two Carers were sent to attend to him with a smile. As time went on myself and the staff developed a sense of humour over this. I would go the staff and say "Sorry folks! He needs positioning for feeding!"

Very quickly two staff would attend to my husband, and I was taken to the front of the queue to be given his lunch as It was crucial to start feeding him as quickly as possible once re-positioned. Then there was the challenge of positioning him again between courses. My golly, they were SO patient and loving with him! "Hello Mr. Brian" they greeted him with or "Hello Handsome Man" and get him laughing and relaxed before moving him. He would be Mr. Grumps while they positioned him once again. All was carried out with a chuckle and trying to make it fun.

As relatives watching our loved one gradually requiring greater care input and manifesting new challenges, it is important to understand the staffs challenges and work "with them" and not "against them". How would we manage twelve hours of attention loving care without even a sign of frustration shown? Those who work in this specialist arena of care are wonderful people who need more recognition than they are given, for what they do on a day to day basis. I think back to when I was coping at home and the days when I was really challenged to stay calm and patient at all times. I watched as staff showed genuine affection for the residents, each with their own unique behaviour patterns. It can be difficult at times to see things from the perspective of a relative as well the staff, but for me this is important to quality care that we so want for the one we love. A team approach may mean acknowledging our own emotional agenda that could influence how we see the caring environment. Learning to accept that, certainly in my own case, the very best is being done for them. Maybe you have been used to doing things a certain way for a long time before your loved one needed nursing care. Watching needs being met in a different way, even with patience and love can bring up frustration and anger. For me, I had to learn to adjust to new routines, new staff, be open to trusting as well as sharing concerns in a positive way. Long term inner emotional programming, even from childhood experiences can easily influence responses during the challenges of your caring and supporting journey. We are all emotional beings and expressing them without guilt or judgement is key to better coping.

Find someone who will listen when you need It. Maybe journal your frustrations and anger or guilt. Consider if you had issues with trust with your parents, sibling or spouse. Acknowledging that this is not an easy road but releasing these emotions, will enable new ways of walking in moments of Inner Peace. My mantra? "I Choose Peace – All is Well in My World". You are grieving loss before the final loss. However, it is essential to find even the smallest of blessings within it. I determined to get on well with the staff to a point where I felt the Care Home was a "second family". Just thanking the staff for their care and praising for making your loved one look great goes a long way along with accepting that little things like – not shaved, hair a mess, no socks or tights on, may just be a non-compliance issue. Mention to the staff and they may well tell you it was a challenging personal care day. Or if not, do what I did and expect a turn around.

I was very happy that somewhere deep down in Brian's brain there was some degree of awareness of myself and other key people who visited along with some of the staff. Some degree of compliance may have been achieved by saying to him "Brian we are going to make you look really nice as your lovely wife is coming to see you soon". I was truly a part of the "nursing unit family" after a short time and the "blip" that took place was just that and I was able to turn the agony of the changes in his condition into having a sense of humour as he became more creative with his restlessness in bed, to help with managing my own emotional responses.

My good and trusty friend along with older sister came to stay regularly and witnessed his antics when we visited. To lighten the situation, I would say as we entered his room, "Look at the state of him today!" And then to Brian "What are we going to do with you? Just Keep Loving You!" As I bent over to give him a hug and kiss – mindful that he might thrash his arms at any moment or mindful he may be Mr. Grumps on that day!

As I look back over the latter stage phase with Brian, my mother's wall plaque comes to mind –

God Grant Me the Serenity
To Accept The Things I Cannot Change
To Change The Things I Can
The Wisdom to Know The Difference

The journey cannot be changed. Even wishing we could turn the clock back will not help. It is all about our decision regarding how we travel the journey.

We have a choice – Victim Mode OR Adaptation and Acceptance.

CHAPTER 4

Conquering with Creativity – Cup of Tea

I was becoming aware of the growing challenges with the late-stage Alzheimer's Disease and the multiplicity of care needs that arise, requiring unique solutions.

My desire to work as a team with the staff enabled the creative spirit to rise up within me, with greater adaptability and acceptance as we grew nearer to the end of the road. It really did seem that way now after over two years, not expecting to carry on his earthly journey with things that transpired (The Rocky Road of 24/7 Care).

Number one adaptation -

It was haircut time again and his hairstyle was becoming difficult to manage, particularly with shampooing. The lovely hairdresser who was gifted with cutting and styling with residents who were not easy to work with, suggested that the best solution for my man was to give him a short haircut. My initial inner response was "Is he going to look like a convict?". I speedily dealt with that and accepted that his care far superseded his hairstyle! Yes, apprehension reared its ugly head when I visited next but the new look actually suited hm! "Oh, you've had your haircut! Love the new style!" I greeted him with and then gave the statutory hug and kiss. He actually laughed as if his awareness and understanding had kicked in for that moment at what I had said. When I asked the hairdresser how the barber session went, she laughed and said, "We managed". I knew that the truth was that Brian was not very compliant and that she would have been very patient with him. It reminded of a situation I witnessed in his previous care unit. There was a lady who was always walking around and never sat still long enough even to get her to eat. It was hair trim day, and it was a case of catch her when you can and have a snip. I jokingly questioned the hairdresser "Is this what you call mobile hairdressing?" So here I am, further getting used to the ongoing high standard of his overall care being given. The new look was definitely in his best interest and would assist in personal care needs being easier for the staff and less stressful for Brian.

Resistance to change in life only serves to increase stress levels and emotional turmoil. The best solution is to accept whilst finding the benefit of the necessary change and not stay in the fear of it.

In this part of my husband's journey, I really needed to pull on that deep Inner Peace available to us all. The mind is so powerful and is always seeking the "status quo". However, how do we learn and develop the courage and strength to keep going if we refuse to embrace fully life's challenges and changes. To be in peace no matter what is an ongoing process throughout life but worth working at. – "I CHOOSE PEACE, ALL IS WELL IN MY WORLD" has been a saving mantra along the way. At the end of the book, you will find my "Five Steps to Inner Peace"

Number two adaptation-

Time to resurrect my sewing skills now, as, dressing Brian in Shirts and Polo Shirts was a huge issue for him, and the staff, who wanted to decrease his stress as much as they could. He had always been independent by nature and liked to do things for himself – while he happily enjoyed my culinary skills each day!! Maybe, with personal care, somewhere deep down in his memory bank he was rejecting interference with personal care intervention from others. There were still moments of awareness manifesting from time to time.

My past skills came in very handy as I deftly carried out my idea – Velcro fastening at the back of his shirts and polos? Yes, you can purchase online but the prices are not exactly bargain!! Out came the sewing machine for an airing and thankfully it still was in good working order. Also, an excuse to go shopping for a new "wardrobe" for him. I always got a buzz out of buying clothing he would have liked to wear before all this set in. I was careful to choose suitable attire for day and night that would not fray during sewing and were colourful along with being laundry friendly. There was a hindsight moment when I thought to myself "Why on earth did I not consider this before!"

For me, I see no reason to neglect the standard of clothing for your loved one because of their diagnosis. If they took a pride in how they dressed prior to their diagnosis, why not continue to take a pride in dressing on their behalf, whilst complying with comfort and practicality.

The staff were overjoyed when I arrived with his new clothing. Routine with Brian was made less stressful for him and the staff, as he became somewhat more compliant, and the routine took less time. I phased in a good supply and replaced as needed.

To be involved where you can with your loved one's care, can be great for assisting with dealing with the roller coaster of emotions as well as give a sense of belonging.

Another "Light Bulb" moment –

This one can be relevant for anyone with a form of Dementia or Alzheimer's Disease, especially if there is a major issue with visual acuity and understanding and comprehension of instructions. They will be fearful in that moment and non-compliant.

It had become evident that plying deodorant to Brian's armpits was not a pleasant experience for him. Cold spray or roll-on deodorant would cause him to cry out and resist. Time for research again! Google came to the rescue with a search in a popular online shopping zone. Listed here were a number of organic, natural, soothing cream deodorants that were kind to the skin. Problem solved and the product worked well for him. This could be a great help when caring for someone or they are in 24/7 care.

Helping Me and Helping Another

Not long after my husband was admitted to Princess Christian Care Home, a lady was admitted to the same unit and immediately "connected" with me. This resulted in my buddying with her husband who, at the same time, formed a great rapport with Brian. He was struggling with his journey, having cared for his wife for a number of years at home. He suggested we go for "tea and cake" on one of the visits and I accepted. We swapped notes and it helped him unwind for a short time. This became an intermittent regularity plus we sometimes shared afternoon tea with our partners in the care home – special cake indulged in courtesy of "buddy". Brian enjoyed interacting with him which was lovely to watch. It was great also, to see his wife's face light up when she saw me and responded to my interactions.

Finding a buddy on this journey can be a big help and support as there is mutual understanding of the emotions of the journey. I valued our little "interludes" especially as my man's condition was changing even more.

Caring for you as a carer is SO important. Finding someone you can chat to on a bad day. Getting to know other relatives in the Care Home and sharing ups and downs and your coping mechanisms, painful moments so that you now that you are not alone. I have found new friends along the way and valued being able to help them as well as receiving encouragement when times have been tough.

No matter how positive I was determined to make this journey and find a purpose from t, it did not prevent me from having to fully participate in it, find ways to overcome emotions which could then help others.

It's amazing what a meet up for a good old English Cuppa, Cake and a Chat will do!!

CHAPTER 5

Awareness or Just Wishful Thinking?

Alzheimer's Disease manifests uniquely with each person it gets a grip on. I watched this over the time that my husband was in the behavioural challenges unit at princess Christian Care Home.

He was admitted due to his being a "sundowner" – awake all night, extremely restless and confused along with increasingly aggressive behaviour outbursts. He had two different personality traits. His cheerful and gregarious make up plus a sudden flip to "naughty neurons" aggression. On admission to the Care Home relatives used to think he might be staff or a relative, so I have been told frequently!

As his disease progressed with the cognitive and speech challenges increasing along with his Posterior Cortex Atrophy taking it's hold, it was as if he was losing any kind of grip he might have on his true self. With communication skills declining, it could be easy to think that he was less aware of what was happening to him. Yet

I have witnessed, right until the end of his life, some degree of awareness. On some of my visiting days he would turn towards me and ask "why?" It was as if at a deep inner level he knew things were not right with him. My response to this was "Only God knows why Brian". Whilst in the previous unit he was on one occasion doing his best to communicate his Barn Dancing times as music played in the background. "I wish we could......." followed by incomprehensible words he told me. It was as if he knew that he was now unable to do what he could before the Alzheimer's Disease began its symptoms. "Never mind, we have our wonderful memories, don't we?" I lovingly responded as I held his hand. He seemed OK with that and was calm through the rest of my visit. Yes, he would go off into what I call "a zone" sometimes, but then return and become aware of people around him. He was always aware of me when I visited- such a blessing!

It is my belief that many people with Alzheimer's Disease have a greater deep inner awareness than we give them credit for. Even the staff agreed with me.

This is why I recommend being careful how you speak around them along with speaking things over them that they will actually hear and comprehend in the moment, which could lead to an "outburst". To illustrate this –

Brian was still spending some of the daytime in his previous unit of care, reclining in his wonderful "banana chair" which I could wheel around to see folks or out into the garden for some fresh air- even if it didn't last long. A slight breeze and he was ready to go back indoors again! On this particular day we were paying a visit to those in the conservatory. During conversation with the head of activities, I very quietly mentioned something from his past that could help with greater understanding of his sudden aggressive and angry outbursts. He was sitting a distance away from us and a loud response came from him "That's right!". Hearing acuity was certainly not an issue! Probably increased due to Posterior Cortex Atrophy manifestations.

That incident taught me a lot. I shared what happened with the staff so that they would be mindful of conversations when caring for him.

During my nursing years, we were constantly reminded of the fact about patients hearing sense- that it is the last sense to go before someone dies or transitions as I call it. We learn of people who recall everything that had been said during their time in a coma. As if true awareness deep within was always present.

Having encountered my husband's underlying awareness made me extra sensitive when family or other friends and relatives visited him. Alzheimer's patients, it seems, are, in essence, no different to other patients/residents and we need to show respect and understanding when interacting with them. One might say that it is possible to come from a point of "wishful thinking" because accepting the changes manifesting with ones loved one is too painful. I do get that; however, for me, I am convinced he had a deep inner awareness that popped up from time to time. Probably his saving grace was that he may well not have retained those moments. Some learnings from this?

- Experience what is happening
- Observe ones reaction for future reference
- Accept the ongoing change
- Look for blessings somewhere amongst it all
- Do the very best to "live in the moment"

In the first few months of his journey in the nursing unit, as I leaned over to give him a hug and a kiss, he tried hard to tell me he loved me plus attempted to wrap his arms around me to return the hug. On one occasion he succeeded and became "locked in" to the point where I looked to see where the emergency bell was situated! I did eventually manage to escape and have a wonderful memory to recall.

Brian definitely had a degree of awareness with some of the staff members when they entered his room to carry out tasks or say hello. His face lit up with a big smile and a laugh that came from a deep sense of knowing.

The lesson here is to err on the side of awareness. Yes, it may well mean being willing to be vulnerable rather than putting up protective barriers that can lead to guilt and regret later on.

In life generally we can have experience of hurt and upset to overcome. Allowing yourself to be vulnerable and seeing those times as something to learn and grow from is the key to finding Inner Peace and Joy through challenging circumstances. It takes work on your part along with determination to overcome in life. It sure is worth it though!

I find it fascinating that science can now show from MRI (magnetic resonance imaging) and PET (positive emission tomography) scans – both show up any abnormality in brain tissue and circulation – brain pathways that stem from a positive attitude to life. Centres in the brain actually I light up when we manifest positive thoughts and express joy and laughter.

In all honesty, there have been moments where I have questioned in my mind just how much deep-down awareness Alzheimer's suffers have. Can some of those outbursts be associated with frustration and anger from past memories along with what they are unable to accomplish in that moment? I decided to deal with the incidents of "awareness manifestation" as they arose, avoiding expressing my own emotions (deal with them after) as they are seemingly "aware" like Brian's "why?" Question.

Then there is the awareness of the Carers in regard to the truth of the journey we take with our loved one. We cannot turn the clock back. Neither can we change what has been. Being aware, as I said earlier, expressing and releasing emotions and letting them go which facilitates acceptance coming to the fore of our mind. Emotional honesty is key to a Carers journey with a loved one whilst not becoming a victim to them.

It was not always easy for me to accept some of my husbands "awareness" moments e.g. The day when he was in the previous unit and with a very sad and downcast expression, he said to me "I think I am losing it down there!". He had been incontinent of faeces and that would continue. I acknowledged it with love without dwelling on it once he had expressed his own feelings. However, I did alert the staff to what had transpired before I left.

So, the overall message here is to be aware of your loved ones "awareness moments", along with being aware of your own self and how you are dealing with each day, seeking help or a listening ear. My listening ear was older sister who I called from the car before leaving for home and making a cup of tea and recalling positive moments or past happy memories.

Rejoice in any positive moments as memories for the future, even if your loved one's awareness expressions do not marry totally with professional opinion. See them as a blessing to recall in the future. This is your journey remember! On my own journey I certainly made a point of capitalising on any "positive awareness" moments and can look back and remember fun times together.

The positive awareness moments are worth treasuring and will help you deal it's with the times when you are getting closer to the end of the road.

CHAPTER 6

Savouring Special Moments

When I look back over the years of our Alzheimer's journey, I am so very thankful that I managed to capture happy moments by photographs and videos, including holidays in the early stages plus some lovely times captured on video during his Care Home stay.

Not long after his admission, relatives were asked to participate in creating Life Story books that would be used by staff as in interaction tool to talk about life memories with the residents. They are also a great diversional therapy instrument to reduce agitation moments. I now have my husbands to keep and browse so that memories stay alive in my mind. How grateful I am for the inventions of iPhone and iPad which enable instant capture and sharing of moments with those who love him but are living at a distance.

When you create those special memories, it can help with dealing with those "if only ...." guilt thoughts that pop up in your mind. With a sense of humour one can have photographs that show a "not so good" day.

Before my husband went up to the full nursing care unit and his condition was progressing, he had many "aggressive moments" that called for extra sensitivity during visits. Even shortening them if necessary to allow the staff to distract him – usually a cup of tea with biscuits did the trick. In the second year following admission our wedding anniversary day had dawned with staff preparing a cake to help us celebrate along with a lovely framed photograph of us both from one of his "happy" days. There was also a singer booked that day and during his entertainment, flowers and chocolates were presented to us. The singer came over and sang especially for us and I was genuinely touched and moved to tears. My man however was not at all impressed and I pondered in my mind what might have been going on deep down inside him. He had been a great folk singer and loved singing and music times in the care home. Was he actually frustrated that his body was not able to do what it had been able? Here I needed a sense of humour around the incident and when I look at the photograph now, I can smile about the day.

In a way, this journey is a reflection of how we deal with life generally. If you look for those special moments in your life from day to day, you are more likely to seek and treasure special moments on this journey, which is SO important for the future.

Instead of being caught up totally in the suffering of Brian, I am, after a few months in from his transition, able to begin to recall moments of joy and times that we laughed together. They compensate hugely for the sad, and painful times.

Depending on how your loved one manifests the Alzheimer's/ Dementia journey, will, of course impact on the number of happy memories you can create along the way. With iPhones and Android phones which we all have these days, it is wonderful way of "snapping" those happy moments. At Princess Christian Care Home, the staff were wonderfully obliging with snapshots and short videos for me! One has to be "quick off the mark" at times or you may, like I did, miss that magic moment! By the time I had got into and set the camera to video to catch his laughter and maybe a few words, the moment had passed. Never mind though, I have some wonderful memories that can be treasured as the Grieving journey and adjustment progresses forward since he "went home".

Life on this earth seems to program us to live in fear of the future, worrying about "supposing...?" What if...?" "Nothing ever goes right with me anyway...". Why not choose to be different and work at looking for the "light in the darkness of grief" – even if it flickers and then goes again. As you begin to actively observe and notice positive moments, it will eventually become a habit. Yes, it takes dedication and determination – I know so from my own life experiences!

Of course, there is pain along this journey knowing the eventual outcome. It takes a process of Acknowledgement, Adjustment and Acceptance as things progress with ones loved one. Following hard work on myself and a decision not to become a total "victim of circumstances", I was able to develop increasing moments of inner peace and do my very best to live "in the moment" – a far cry from someone who in their twenties "crossed bridges" in life months ahead! I am reflecting on the Care Home journey with my husband as I write, realising how blessed I was to know that he was in excellent hands with the staff. I could leave from my visits to deal with any emotions I needed to be at peace and sleep at night. That, of itself, is a happy memory.

It is also beneficial to you as the carer, to create some joyous moments for you without feeling guilty. It will help with later adjustment to creating your own life as you grieve their transition. Have the courage (or face the fear and do it anyway!) to go out with trusted friends and family. People who will do their best to understand where you are at and uplift and encourage. Share with them ANY positive moments and those you have found humour in so that you begin to embed them in your memory bank.

I recall one Sunday morning at church following my husband's transition where the last song was "How Great Thou Art", a hymn we had at our wedding, and I also chose for his ashes internment. Interestingly as we are singing, my mind immediately took me back to his internment day where I stood looking at his box of ashes. Yes, I had a grieving moment with tears and a hug from one of the ladies. I then laughed and said" God could have shown me the wedding memory instead!" Having carried out that exercise, it then became easier to recall the celebration part of the internment of ashes as Members of his Barn Dance Band played music and we had fun attempting some dances. It was lovely to recall some of the fun times we had enjoyed during his "calling" days. As I write, it is less emotional as I look back to that day.

So, the message here is –

- Practice, practice, practice creating and treasuring the good moments with your loved one.

- Practice creating some joyous moments for You to help as you move into creating a new norm for your life.

<u>CHAPTER 7</u>

The Last Hurdle

This journey is very much like facing hurdles. I had faced and dealt with many hurdles on this our new journey, from the early days right up until right now. As I reflect back, I am genuinely amazed at how I have adapted to each new phase of my husband's journey.

So, here we are, at yet another hurdle and over four years in his 24/7 care. This phase is going to test my ability to create Inner Peace and come to terms with knowing that this is indeed the final part of his journey.

We have come through not expecting him to make it to the three previous Christmas's! Yet somehow, he is managing to be around for yet another one and be able to be aware of favourite cousins visiting, and my Sister recently over the Christmas period.

He is now on his second round of antibiotics for dysphasia and aspiration related chest infections, where food and fluids can trickle down to the lungs. He is, however seeming to respond to them well. Due to his overall condition, it was decided to treat Christmas Day as any other day and be with him as per usual for a visit, whilst indulging in our own festive lunch which was presented on trays beautifully decorated with a Christmas decoration. No detail spared as always! Brian – appetite still at peak performance – had pre-mash Christmas dinner and his favourite thickened Mango juice. One was extra careful with feeding and on high alert for a coughing fit as he struggled at times to swallow. This meal, however, went relatively well with only a minor coughing fit.

It was a blessing that he was aware of both mine and sisters' presence. The staff, who were extremely sensitive to his condition, also treated the day as any other day of the year. Music was kept to quiet and soothing Christmas music along with other music sourced from the internet, specific to healing and relaxation. This did have the effect of minimising agitation episodes.

This was not my moment to treasure. Used to being able to spend time with my man, give hm a hug, and knowing that this time it definitely would be his last Christmas. Time now to practice really being "in the moment", know he is experiencing incredible care in a wonderful environment, be able to rest overnight back at home.

Inner self discussions began to take place as to how I would tackle the final stage. Would I crumble and become a grieving, emotional wreck over what I knew could very soon be happening? By now I had turned to my belief in a supportive God and took comfort from some verses in the "good book", as I often call the bible. For example, there is a verse in the New Testament where Jesus says – "My Peace I leave with you...let not your heart be troubled, neither let it be afraid". Hmm, ties in with Mantra that also had helped me through "I choose Peace – All IS Well in My World". So, there is a Peace we can call on in times of trouble and stress to support us. A Peace from a higher source.

Another verse that has helped is from the New Testament also – "Casting All your Care on Him (Jesus), for he cares for You". Whether you have a belief in God or not, repeating these verses can be a great help in generating Inner Peace.

A decision worth making that will help carry you through difficult times is to work at "being at peace" no matter what. Oh! Yes! It has to be worked at and practiced regularly along with acknowledging the importance of expressing sorrow during the most challenging time of the Alzheimer's journey – letting go. What is not helpful to anyone is to remain in abject sorrow continuously when some degree of Inner Peace is attainable.

So, Christmas passes, and my husband seems reasonably comfortable – fidgeting, laughing, eating and drinking, when yet again a chest infection develops with more antibiotics necessary. Coughing fits were becoming more common now, so a second referral request is made for a visit from the specialist nurse at the local hospital. Confirmation of his puréed diet and thickened fluids to grade four takes place.

In spite of the chest infection challenge, Brian has moments of awareness and tries to say something, offering a happy sound as the statutory visiting hug takes place.

As I watched subtle ongoing changes take place, I made a conscious decision not to focus solely on what I could see was ahead. Instead, I focused on ensuring as much as was possible, my man had awareness of my presence on the regular visits that took place. I also had to make a decision to tell myself that I was doing the very best I could and not allow guilt to take hold plus keep holding on to my belief that he would be going to a better place with his spirit when the time came for him to transition.

It was by now, May/June of 2019 with Sisters regular summertime visit taking place. She noticed a big change in Brian, in spite of the fact that he knew her voice and recognised her touch along with being able to respond to her chats with him. What had been interesting was that prior to her coming down, I had kept saying to him "Maureen is coming to visit soon" and he would give a big grin and utter "Oh!". Food is still a pleasurable experience for him, as well as we could have times where he would laugh with us. When staff entered his room, he seemed to recognise voices as they used their standard greeting "Hello Mr Brian" or "Hello Handsome Man". It was a joy to see how they interacted with him. My opinion is that the majority of Carers really do care from the heart. I had many a fun interaction with the staff and they kept me up to date on Brian at each visit.

It is beneficial to keep a rapport with the staff and be able to get a full picture of your loved one's day to day condition. Not being concerned about approaching them will help as they are "busy bees" and will happily talk with you – I found this so at Princess Christian care Home.

Yes, in many ways, one was going through inner pain at watching my man suffer yet free of pain and maintaining his longstanding appetite. It was a sad day when he managed to whisper to me "Why, Why?"; as if deep down somewhere he knew that things were not as they used to be. My best answer I could muster was "We don't know why darling. Only God knows why" which seemed to calm him down. Past self- talk on this journey came to mind then – "Sylvia, this is Brian's journey. You cannot do it for him. Just love him and be there for him."

That is the very best you can do for a loved one. I often say that no matter what research takes place, no one will get into the mind of someone walking the Dementia/Alzheimer's path.

CHAPTER 8

Saying Goodbye

In many ways, on the Alzheimer's journey you are saying goodbyes all the way through – all part of the process of Acknowledge, Accept and Adjust I wrote about earlier. Then comes the eventual, final physical adjustment process as the spirit gets ready to fly.

My dear man became victim to yet another aspiration chest infection and this time in spite of two courses of antibiotics there was no improvement. I said to the staff that a third try could take place with a review following. This could well be when I had to face the final physical "goodbye".

However, one may succeed to adaptation to change, however strong one's belief in a higher power, however strong a belief that you will see them again in spirit form for eternity, this part of the journey is challenging.

The doctor's day to visit dawned a few days after the decision to try one more dose age of antibiotics, which had not made impact and I was asked to go and see the Head Nurse of his unit. Even now, as I write, I am recalling this time again, but I want to help you, the reader, receive hope from how saying goodbye can be a time of joy amongst the sorrow of having no more physical contact.

The doctor had recommended it was time to stop all medication and let Brian enjoy food and fluids as he desired whilst keeping him comfortable. I agreed to this. He was, I knew, in the most amazing care environment for this final stage of his journey. He was put on their "red alert" scheme with half hourly checks and monitoring for any sign of pain or discomfort.

Being blessed with strong support from my sister in Scotland a dear friend in Lincolnshire, who Brian was still aware of, I alerted them to the current situation. Their love for my husband and wonderful support kicked in instantly. The next day my dear friend arrived, and by the Friday Sister arrived from Scotland.

On your journey, please try your utmost to obtain some trustworthy support and allow folks to give that. People do want to care and show love in this world. Just make sure that you still walk your journey on your terms as you allow constructive "organising "of you. At this time, emotions tend to go somewhat crazy and what I call "grass hopping" with day to day tasks can very easily take place.

It was time for practicality to kick in at home - organising sleep zones, extra food supplies. My two adorable cats would naturally relish in extra fuss and attention! My responsibility here? Don't allow any spoiling I have to deal with at a later date!

With immediate plans in place, I knew my man would want to see his favourite cousins as much as they would wish to see him also at this time of saying goodbye. I told Brian that he was going to have visitors. His usual response was forthcoming – a smile and "ahh". Incredibly it was as if deep down awareness seemed to be evident with him.

Myself, sister and friend were in agreement to spend as much time with Brian as possible – we did not know how many days he would stay with us.

A routine was set up for visiting which included a night shift and each of us taking turns to get some sleep. The staff were wonderful and set up a room for us to use and invited us to feel at home and make drinks as we wished in between their provisions for us. We took it in turns to get three hours sleep each – me first, second sister followed by friend.

So – first night! This was an interesting experience! I took first turn and as I laid on what was a "super firm" mattress, suddenly ripples began to go up my back and down again, subsiding for a few seconds and then repeating. I was trying to get some sleep on an air mattress! "How do residents adjust and get a good night's sleep" I said to myself. We had a good laugh at the first night's sleep attempts with the units head nurse. Bless them, by that evening they had exchanged the air mattress for a regular mattress. It was standard practice in the nursing unit for all residents to have an air mattress on their bed.

Breakfast was offered – eggs, beans and sausages with pots of tea and toast on trays. It was like being in a hotel!

Brian was now enjoying chocolate flavoured Forti creme mousse along with favourite Mango juice as his staple diet administered by extremely patient and understanding staff members.

Red alert checks were diligently carried out and personal care routines continued with his Velcro fastening polo shirts for clothing. No detail was spared in their care for him. Nothing was too much trouble for him and us too.

Knowing he was getting such wonderful care, our daily routine for the first few days was to stay till around 1pm, have a break and return around 7pm for overnight vigil. We had a couple of nights where we stayed till around 1am and then went home for some quality rest as they would call if anything changed – fortunately I live only ten minutes' drive from the Care Home. My prayer had been that I could be with him up to his last physical breath, unless he wished to transition alone. Some folks choose to do this.

Painful as this final part of the journey is, it is very important to consider their needs above anything else while caring for you. Allow support from caring and understanding people around you but still remember this is your journey. Understandably, for some, they cannot cope with the final phase and will not be able to keep up the vigil that we chose to do. Preferring to rely on the staff care, plus phone calls if they need to visit either before they transition or following that moment. Whatever your choice is endeavour to carry it through in a way that eliminates guilt and "if only's" at a later date. I have witnessed many "if only's" during my career in nursing which can be emotionally destructive. Everything in life is about choice. Your choices with your loved one have and are being made. The outcome of choices is what they are and new choices can then be made that will serve you better as you learn from them. My choice around the last couple of weeks with my husband does not mean I judge those who make a different choice. Circumstances differ with all of us, and we respond to life in a variety of ways. Most of all tapping into the Inner Peace will help us through.

As the days passed and Brian's life here was drawing to a close, it was awesome to see the loving care taking place, with staff from his previous unit coming up to see him, daily visits from the Home Manager, activities team and other departments with their jolly greeting - "Hello my friend" from the Manager, "Hello Mr Brian" or "Hello handsome man" from staff and activities team. Most times he would muster up a smile of recognition. This was a very moving scene to witness as well as a lovely memory for us.

There can be some moments to treasure amongst the emotional roller coaster times.

As the days and nights continued, a decision was made to set up a syringe driver (a way of continuously dripping into his system calming medication and prevent fluid from building up in his lungs) to make him comfortable. Thankfully he was not showing any signs of being in pain. The management of the very last days were amazing.

We took turns at sitting close to him and making contact – holding his hand and gently stroking his forehead, which he liked, along with talking to him as we normally would until he took his last breath.

The very worst thing that can take place at this stage, or any stage of the Dementia's journey, is "talking over your loved one". Their hearing will be acute right up until their journey ends. The hidden awareness that may well show from time to time should be taken to consideration. Brian's awareness popped up regularly in the final stages.

Happy memories were talked about with joy and humour whilst his relaxing music played for him in the background or some of his favourite folk and barn dance tunes.

As the end time grew closer, it was time to encourage him to let his spirit fly heavenward. Because of our spiritual belief I could tell him that Jesus was waiting for him, along with reassurance that I and family were OK and would be absolutely fine.

The Well-being staff member introduced a calming diffuser into his room and gave him hand massages which one could see he enjoyed.

On the day we said farewell to physical Brian I spent a while with him on my own chatting and reassuring him that our love was God given and eternal. This took courage but is something that assisted a calm and peaceful transition.

Doing this with a loved one can be a beautiful moment plus, for some, a healing time as you express regrets if You have any or ask forgiveness. Many a relationship has been healed during the last few days of the patient's life which facilitates a peaceful passing and relief for their loved one.

With the very special end of life care carer present with us, Brian peacefully took his last two breaths later that day.

CHAPTER 9

Celebrate!

Expecting my man to go home two years previously had set in motion basic preparations. He had expressed a desire to be cremated so I chose a beautiful natural burial ground not too far from home and a plot by a lake where I could visit and sit and reflect or do some writing with a picnic and flask. Opportunity also to recall the wonderful times we had, even during his time of care at Princess Christian Care Home.

His funeral would be a life celebration and of all he had given to humanity whilst here on earth. Dedication in his role as a sales representative in the "kitchens to builders" industry, always going the extra mile for his customers. The joy he brought to thousands over a 31-year period of heading up and calling for the Stockbrokers Belt Barn Dance Band. Very apt for the Surrey County!

The Life Celebration took place at the natural burial ground as part of his ashes internment ceremony. The Minister conducted a great, short service with a life story video including Brian singing in the background that was really moving to all. He gave great encouragement to us about the life following death and where Brian now was in his new spiritual body. I knew that I would meet my man again one day in a body free of disease and suffering. Probably enjoying barn dancing in heaven!

Some of his original band members attended and played music for us. After the buffet was finished, it became time to fully celebrate the wonderful gift of joy he gave to so many.

The guitarists wife became caller as we organised ourselves into a typical "longways set". Music started and we followed instructions for one of his favourite and popular dances that is supposed to be easy to do! Being afternoon time, all minds should be sharp and able to easily follow the callers' instructions. Sure enough there was much laughter as mistakes were made and I knew that we were not "in sync" with the music. No different to the many fun evenings with the punters while here on earth. "He's probably looking in on us and wanting to sort things out" I said with a laugh to the dancers!

If you have any belief in an afterlife available for humanity, then death of the physical body is a celebration of a spirit body that is alive and well. This was uppermost in my mind at this time, and I felt a sense of joy about his freedom and our meeting again.

How pleased I was that prior planning had been put in place, including his life movie enabling other essentials to be take care of with minimal stress and anxiety. The support I received from the Care Home plus sister and long-standing friend was great as we arranged the life celebration practicalities and short funeral service.

This is a very emotional time, and the initial shock of a loved one passing can make you very vulnerable. If you have chosen to organise a simple "goodbye" then stick to your plan and don't allow yourself to get coerced into arrangements that are more costly than what was originally decided. Remember that the people helping you are also running a business. During my Care Management days, I witnessed cases of emotional manipulation resulting in extra costs to the grieving loved ones.

When organising a simple buffet for my husband's life celebration, I was challenged and had to stand my ground. "Oh, but when people come back from the ashes internment, they like to have a glass of wine!". No, we did not want alcohol in the early afternoon plus most of the people attending would be driving. An internet search came up with a simple buffet that met our requirements.

Following the short crematorium service, the Care Home put on wonderful spread for us and a favourite photograph of Brian set in the midst. Staff and residents relatives came down to offer their condolences. It was like being with my "other family" who really cared for both of us. With much food left over, it was a pleasure to share it between the units for the staff and residents. The lovely music, golden "treble clef" floral tribute was placed in the Care Home's small memorial garden to bring colour for a while.

This care home certainly knows how to support relatives at this time and I am pleased to be part of the "family". Yes, I am still in as much contact as possible and part of their "friends of Princess Christian" to this day.

SO. How does one move forward after the long journey?

PART 2

The Pathway Towards Peace and Purpose

CHAPTER 1

Reflections and Moving On

How does one move on from a long journey with a loved one - watching the changes, their suffering and frustrations?

For me there was a relief, whilst knowing I had to get used to visiting the Care Home without my man to support any more. Adjusting to acceptance that he was in a better place. Knowing that with our belief in a heaven, I will see him again and spend eternity with him. It also made me have empathy for those who do not believe in any form of life after death, making the transition of their loved one an extremely painful experience as they deal with what is for them, absolute finality.

Even if one believes in a spiritual body that lives on, coupled with the joy of seeing them again, the physical contact is going to be missed and be a journey of adaptation.

During the journey there is ongoing dealing with constant change – behaviour, for some, not being recognised any more, gradual loss of their ability to do anything for them-self to needing everything done for them.

I was indeed blessed that my man had awareness of me right until the day he transitioned into the arms of Jesus.

What do I miss most as I pen this chapter? Having a bear hug and "I love you darling!"

Moving on from the passing of a loved one does not mean we block out the past but create the lovely memories and let the moments of "If only I could...." Express themselves and then override with a happy experience or a memory that counteracts the emotions of the moment.

I was chatting with a lady at church who told me that it is four years since her husband passed away, and she still misses the physical touch from time to time, as much as she knows she will see him again. I do not resonate with those who say, "You will get over it!". I would rather speak of adjusting to a new life – new experiences. Growing into a person who can build a new life interspersed with memories. Building a new emotional agenda for yourself as you let the rocky road of past emotional expressions drift slowly away and work towards a sense of Inner Peace and Joy. Notice that I said work.

This moving forward journey has its own challenges and takes time to adjust to it. For me, there is an importance to finding out that peace and joy are an inner experience that resides deep in your spirit being to help override the feelings of sorrow and loss – the guilt, denial, anger and grief, overpowering grief.

Moving on can be described as another emotional roller coaster of adjustment and acceptance as you release your loved one to be free of suffering and healed in a new spirit body. Or if you do not have the same belief that I do, being able to close the curtains and treasure past memories or deal with releasing past regrets. Having photographs around the home that help you recapture the life you had with them prior to their condition. Talk to their photo and let out those feeling that rise up about them having left you to cope with everything. I sometimes wake up in the morning and say, "Hello Handsome in Heaven!" And then move into the day's activities.

The pain of not being able to do things with them, or sudden change of the "usual" routine will rise up – even not having Care Home visits which had become part of "normal routine". Practicing to deliberately override the pain with a happy time does help. I recall coming home from a Care Home visit one day and being in a very emotional state, I did some self- talk and made a cup of tea, sat down at the dining room table, wept for a full minute and then, with effort, closed my eyes and recalled our beautiful wedding day. Yes, it worked! The emotional pain subsided, and I could then get on with the rest of my day. I recommend doing this, creating your own experience, when those grief emotions hit hard. Grieving positively does take effort and determination. You are transitioning into a "new normal" and it hurts.

Christmas is looming after Brian transitioned in the September and I attended the church carol service with my sister. As I sang one of the carols – husband's favourite – tears began to flow, but I kept on singing through the tears as I imagined him there with me. A sense of peace began to flood through me and ease the pain.

I am fully realising as time goes on, that this "moving on" really is like moving to a new country and adjusting to their culture difference. It will be different for many depending on how life was previously and how you have reacted to life's experiences. Whatever your situation was, this IS a new road you are travelling. A personal map has to be created to assist. Creating that map will involve accepting that as emotions arise, you will go off track at times and may need to have a "pit-stop" and review of the emotions that are coming up within you. Part of that review will be an honest approach to expressing them.

- Are they linked with past ways of dealing with change in life?
- Is there guilt or anger rising? – the "What if I had just ...? Or "Why did they have to leave me right now?"
- "How am I going to survive without them?"

How you and your loved one related to each other overall, will impact the "new norm" emotional responses and adjustment process.

I feel blessed that I have been able to support a man who loved unconditionally, and in his own wonderful way, showed that love right up to his "transition day'. I had to tell him he was OK for his spirit to move on and that I would be fine. Turning sorrow in to solutions has been my calling from my journey, and so I will continue to do.

Can you turn life's experiences into something to help others? I heard a powerful speaker once say "If you are going through a difficult time, find a way to help someone else. It will gladden your heart and help you overcome".

As I look back, I realise the amazing learning curve I have been going through. In spite of a successful nursing career, care management involving dementia patients, along with Master Coaching skills and a spiritual faith, I still had to deal my own emotions on the Alzheimer's journey with my husband. I had to bring together all my other life experiences and what I had learned into play to generate a greater emotional balance. They were crucial to the rocky road of emotions that manifested.

In reality, anyone on their Dementia's journey with a relative, is having a life experience that can be a learning and growing time or living as a victim to it. Becoming an emotional wreck without seeking to deal with the emotional roller coaster can definitely have an impact on physical health and wellbeing. Science can now conclusively show how our thoughts influence Brain tissue with a release of hormones and chemicals into the bloodstream that wreak havoc in the body system functions.

For me, it became a choice to ride the emotional roller coaster in a way that would lead to greater emotional stability with an attitude that could generate a positive and calm response to life. It is still a work in progress and will be so until I decide to transition from my physical body. As I move on with my new pathway and calling, my desire is to help others from my own life schooling.

You too, as a Carer, have the opportunity, with effort, to either become victorious over your emotions, or to stay in emotional victimhood.

How do you do that you may ask? By facing up to the emotions as they rise up, seek out the trigger. Then you can create new ways to view what is happening. No, it is not an instant cure! However, as you succeed once and celebrate, you have a blueprint for future times.

Over time I have come to realise that there is a greater power that will help us through life – I call him God –, and in his "book" there are some verses of scripture to help us lean on his power. Fact or fiction for you as a reader, Jesus taught us that He will give us Peace. In the gospel of John chapter 14 v 17 he says "Peace I leave with you, my peace I give unto. Not as the world give I unto you. Let not your heart be troubled, neither let it be afraid". It has been a great source of comfort to me. Another scripture I have found helpful from the New Testament 1Peter chapter 5 v 7(A V) is "Casting the whole of your care (all your anxieties, all your worries, all your concerns, once and for all) on Him for He cares for you. Meaning, give Jesus all your cares and swap for his Inner Peace.

What a great exercise to use to help in difficult times. Combined with dealing with your emotional trigger points, can result in a more balanced walk-through challenging time. Yes, it takes consistent dedication and I still daily offload care and seek Inner Peace. Especially as I pen this book during the 2020 COVID 19 with all its challenges.

Why not choose to do Your caring Journey differently than many do?

When you have a more balanced way of looking at what is going on with your caring journey, it will enable you to be more confident with objectively standing your ground when you need to and to keep on fighting to see the right outcomes that you know should be taking place. Whether it be – care input – respite care – letting go and accepting 24/7 care for your loved one – accessing funding assistance etc.

I have learned that by being at peace wherever possible with greater emotional balance throughout the Alzheimer's journey, does not include a passive "no point in asking" or "no point in pursuing" outlook.

A calm and positive approach (needs working on you to achieve whenever possible) to living life and the caring journey, will bring courage and persistence when needed, that facilitates the very best care for your loved one.

- An understanding when things aren't right
- An appreciation of Why things aren't right
- An objective persistence to gain the right outcome

So I finish with this:-

- Recognise when you are emotionally fragile
- Deal with it
- Generate Inner Peace and Joy
- Persist in creating your own emotional balance
- Persist in creating a caring journey that serves you well along with the one being cared for

Looking back, my journey was a daily readjustment of emotions and acceptance along with facing up to situations that needed an objective approach rather than a victim mentality, to facilitate the best outcome possible in that moment.

One huge thing I am learning right now – four to five months since my husband's passing, is to pace myself! There are days when I need to focus on essential tasks and rest. A great grief specialist and Minister based in the United States, suggests doing just three important things each day as you progress with the "new life" journey.

However positive one may wish to be as the "moving forward" journey progresses, grief moments hit you hard. For me it is "If only I could give him a hug". My belief that I will be with him again one day, does provide some comfort during these moments or even days. However, I would not wish him back to suffer as he had done. I have a large teddy bear in the house which I decided to use as my Brian Hug bear. He has a small key ring picture place around his neck and when I need a hug, I cuddle him and have taken him to bed with me for comfort.

What can you create to help on Your journey?

We have to find a way to "let our loved one go" and focus on good times, or if life with your loved one was not as great as you would have wished for, make a decision to release the "I wish" and any accompanying guilt and tell oneself that you forgive the past and will work at adjusting to your changed world.

Why not write a letter to them or talk to a photograph or whatever expression suits your personality? As sad and painful emotions seem ever to rear themselves in the mind it is OK to acknowledge them, express them but not make them the only focus, becoming a chronic "victim" of circumstances.

Feeling sorrow after a loved one has transitioned is normal but staying in the sorrow every single moment can impact on overall health and wellbeing. Every one's grief journey is unique and cannot be put in a "grief" box. The ten steps grief process so widely known about can, when taken as definite stages to follow, it may surprise you when you find that you are not following them like a straight road. For example, where you stop at the "shock" traffic lights for a while, move on to the "emotional release" traffic lights and then the "anger" lights and so on until you celebrate the destination of acceptance.

Grief can take on the most incredible roller coaster ride that is unique to you. Those of you reading who have cared for a loved one with a chronic illness and particularly the Dementia's journey will have been engaging in painful grieving moments as you watch your loved one disappearing in front of your eyes while they are still alive here on earth.

As time went on with my lovely man and his Alzheimer's neuron deterioration took place I was grieving and adjusting almost daily. If this is you, then you, like me may well have had that initial sense of relief and joy that they are free of suffering. Then as time goes on the loss of any form of physical touch hits hard at frequent intervals.

How have I chosen to deal with that? rejoice in him being free of his journey of suffering along with honouring him for allowing his suffering to be turned into a calling to help other Carers on their "Emotional Roller Coaster ride".

<u>CHAPTER 2</u>

Not What I Expected

It is almost six months on since Brian's transition and, in spite of all I learned on the journey, plus what I have created to help others, it is like I have been hit by a train or "my get up and go just got up and went!". You do all that needs to be done, funeral etc. Deal with the snail pace of the UK Probate system as COVID 19 kicks in, initiate a retrospective appeal for the full funding he should have received, and suddenly the pain of not having him here in the physical to hug and tell him I love him kicks in. From a spiritual perspective, you give this care up to God and feel a sense of peace run through you.

Then suddenly, for no reason, tears are flooding down and there cannot be a rational explanation for them. "Why am I feeling like this? I know he is in heaven, and I will see him again!". Then, a realisation dawns that there is no point in questioning- just allow the grief to rise and slowly fade as inner peace begins to kick in once more.

You wake up in the morning, your body feels like it has the Flu, albeit you are not really "feeling ill". OK, the day will be somewhat different as the body demands extra rest and adjustments to daily tasks. The mind cries out" I should be *doing things*. Then a little Google search tells you that grieving takes time – *allow yourself time, be kind to you. Grief Will hit you from time to time over the years, focus on memories that uplift you.*

I recall chatting to someone at church whose husband had transitioned four years previously. She still had his favourite shirt hanging in the wardrobe. Stroking it from time to time gave her a sense of his love being with her.

The conversation with a neighbour gives a sense of hope that you will carry on. He is motoring home in a beautiful red Morgan Convertible car. His story - "I was promised this back in the 1990's by my father who was as excited as I was about the car. After purchasing, I was looking forward to him enjoying a drive out with me. It didn't happen because he suddenly died just before I bought it. Recently whilst driving, I was hit by the grief of not fulfilling that dream with him. I had to pull into a lay-by as the tears streamed down my cheeks for a few minutes.

Moving on from caring for someone for so long – watching bits of them slowly disappear before your eyes is so confusing. You have that sense of relief that they aren't suffering whist missing the routine of visits to see them in the Care Home. You have adjusted to being in the house alone. The two adorable cats are great company. It is not about wishing him back in that body which so awfully suffered as a brain became more and more strange in its function. The times when the deep-down sense of awareness kicks in and he whispered "Why?" With my response "We will never know why darling. Only God knows why". Tears flow as you feel their long journey of suffering as if it is yours, when you learned how to cope with changing behaviours and agonisingly watch the slow deterioration over the years. Such a cruel disease! The happy moments surface and you feel better until – the next grief moment hits you hard.

I had vowed I would not sorrow as the earthly mind does but lean totally on God and his reassuring passages of Scripture. You do that, remembering those written about who wept bitterly during their life including Jesus. Grief is part of the earthly life during adjustment to a new expression of day to day living.

When our heart has been so deeply wounded and crushed, emotional healing has to take place. Just like an open wound, people's healing time is not predictable. That person was a part of you – whether deeply loved or with regret concerning how you wished it could have been.

It is important that you express grief and grow through the process. Someone shared with me. – "My father died over a year ago and I just got on with life, thinking I was doing really well. then not long after the first year had passed, the deep loss hit me, Wham!"

Please don't avoid grieving and grieving in your own way. We are all unique individuals who respond to painful circumstances differently. Grieving helps release those painful emotions positively and cause less impact on one's physical health.

The key thing to moving on and adjusting gradually to a new life is to allow the grieving moments to rise up, release them, which facilitates the healing process to do its work.

CHAPTER 3

Being True to My New Life Journey

No matter how much I tapped into my "Inner Peace" belief, I was determined to participate in a new journey of "grieving well".

The physical loss and heart wrenching feeling slammed into me one morning and I sobbed as the realisation kicked in that the physical contact was to be no more. No more hugs and being able to hold his hand with some acknowledgement from him during the last weeks of his earthly life. I was now not any different to others grieving the loss of a loved one. The pain was real and had to be worked through. No escaping the adjustment to a new way of life.

- Learning to keep memories alive with joy instead of sorrow.
- Learning to adjust to being one instead of two - for me a "widow"

- Learning to understand that there will be folks around you who don't "get it".
- Learning to accept that my grief journey will be unique to me
- Learning to talk about the Alzheimer's journey in dealing with probate etc and acknowledging being a widow
- Learning to allow this journey to empower me in some way that can be used to help others
- Learning to deal with the challenges of essentials such as Pension adjustment, Probate, deciding whether or not to continue appealing for retrospective full care funding.

I found that in the beginning I was keeping myself SO busy, it was as if I wanted to avoid those moments of grief and feeling of loss. It was when the moment of deep sorrow hit me that I decided to do my very best to balance each day with self- care as best I could, while dealing with the government systems that were slower than normal due to the COVD restrictions. I had a great support with my Sister in particular, who let me express those moments of challenge with emotions alongside the practical issues I was facing.

When grieving, to do the journey well, you need to find a support person that is totally unconditional and doesn't try to "fix you". So often we hear about "getting over" grief and "getting on with life". Of course, life does move on, and I was learning that it would be different and only fully understood by myself.

Even with the support folks around me, I was determined to walk through this new emotional trek. The memories that were foremost in my mind were of his most troublesome suffering during the last eighteen months of his life. Happy memories seemed so far away and inaccessible. Looking at photographs didn't even help.

All I would see in my mind were images associated with painful memories. It was almost a year following his transition before I could muster up happy memories in amongst the sad ones. If only I could fully understand what he really suffered. I suppose, in my own way, I was trying to rationalise the whole journey, when deep down in my spirit I knew that it wasn't in my power to try to explain all that he had gone through – just to know that I had no reason to wonder if anything could have gone better.

As soon as the happy memories began to surface, I wanted to share them. Strangely, I had to give myself permission to talk about my dear man. There seemed to be a challenge with the balance of moving on whilst keeping his love and memory alive. Maybe I was not wanting to feel the pain of missing him? How I empathise with those travelling their own unique grief pathway.

It has become clear to me, that if one can accept that it may all seem as if one is looking for a way out of the forest of confusion; each tree represents a different manifestation of emotional response; the forest a winding pathway, seemingly like a maze with no clear exit.

If you, reader, are in your "grief forest" right now, I understand totally. Dealing with the emotions you're going through, could be like going up to the emotional tree, hugging it and facing the emotion followed by replacing with I have talked about earlier in the book. Like absorbing energy from the rising sap in the tree.

As I have travelled through my own emotional forest, I can, as I write, see the value in expressing emotions but not allowing them to totally consume you, and staying there. A bit like hugging the one tree and ignoring the others that link to the way forward to the sunlight as the forest gradually fades behind you.

For me, I felt deep sorrow at his suffering, the "I want a hug", frustration that he missed out on the available funding, the joy I had in buying clothes for him and lovingly altering them for his comfort. Even purchasing a special deodorant cream for his personal care routine. Also interesting, is that the happy memories are overridden with the day-to-day life challenges, that cause you to project your emotions through them.

It was a great day when I could look at the photographs of happy times and smile and not cry. Turning the emotional turmoil from deep pain to being able to remember those happy time's together without regret takes time and will vary with each individual; depending on how you respond to life's challenges generally – the glass half full or half empty.

So don't beat yourself up if the deep pain of it all doesn't fall into a specific timescale for adjustment. Just know that you can and will adjust to your new life, dealing with those emotional trees that pop up to be hugged when it happens.

Well, here I am with a new title to accept and add to those drop-down menus. As far as I am concerned, I am still Brian's wife – after all his spirit is still alive and well! OK, I have to say I am officially a Widow now. Interesting how that takes time to come to terms with, along with telling officials and others that he died a year ago. I decide to capitalise on my new title – it seemed to generate genuine empathy when dealing with tradesmen and unwanted phone calls. Getting removed from "lists" without long conversations was easy!

Every situation of change in life is an opportunity to accept and adjust. It may be painful during the process as emotions want to fight change. Throughout my life I have battled with different situations, only finding peace and contentment by going through the change process, acknowledging the emotional pain experienced, whilst moving forward and emerging to a new way of looking at life.

Fear of change is natural to human beings. We love our "comfort zone". So, understandably, when something like the passing of a loved one hits hard and adjustment to a new unknown world, it is majorly scary to face up to. But it has to be faced. The best decision in a time of confusion and emotional agony, is to face the fear, with support of a trustworthy persons/s one step at a time and allow for gradual inner peace to rise up along with courage to keep going. Let me say here and now, I have had years of practice with numerous "grief" situations arising in my life. It's that old saying "it's not What happened but your response to what happened".

One year has now passed as I continue to adjust to my title of "widow" and the "grief bursts" that come unexpectedly. I tell folks "Well, I have done my first year now." As I expect somewhere in my mind, a magic wand to wave that says – "Now I move on, and all grieving is done!". It also seems that the world around you expects you to "move on" - you've done all the major anniversaries!

Huh! It's not quite like that. This is someone on the road of grieving with its sudden Grief potholes that pop up to be dealt with. As those grieving, it's necessary to appreciate that those who have not been where you are, will not "get it" that sad moments and sad days are quite "normal". The essential thing to realise is that when these "grief potholes" arise, they can be circumnavigated by allowing emotions to be expressed and the pothole filled with positive memories and gratitude that you are travelling well on your journey of adjustment. Celebrate the good days and always remember to continue to take good care of You.

My new road will look different to yours. Keep in your thoughts that "Everyone's grief journey IS Unique to Them".

After around fourteen months I am just beginning to find that the grief potholes are not appearing as frequently – I had many to deal with on the Alzheimer's journey. For me, it is because I do believe in Jesus and the Peace he offers; along with moving over the years, from a glass half empty to a glass half full. I feel blessed to have been a part of Brian's life and the unconditional love he gave me. It was a joy to support him throughout his Alzheimer's journey.

Your new pathway may suddenly come in front of you. You may not be able to see a way to step on to it. If you are trying to move forward and adjust, the pathway may look like nothing but those grief potholes ahead. That's OK. One step at a time with those feet which seem almost too heavy to lift and acknowledge the pain. It is normal as part of grieving. Don't try to compare yourself to others or the almost "linear" grief stages model. So long as you are making baby steps it is OK. Babies never walk initially without falling and having to get up again.

If you feel really stuck and unable to keep moving forward, seek support from someone you can trust or professional support to help you and be there for you. remember the Tools for release – tears, write to your loved one and then destroy, talk with your trustworthy support, use creative skills to express. Some of the famous artists were putting their emotions on canvas. You can play music that reminds you of a moment of joy. I enjoy playing a favourite hymn from our wedding day and singing with gusto, sometimes through tears. It helps!

How about a walk-in nature or by water – the ocean calls me. This can be very calming and create a sense of peace. If you have a spiritual belief or belief in God, bundle them up and give them to him in exchange for his peace. Most of all do what resonates best with you and take your time adjusting to a new way of life.

Many grieving individuals have created something to help others as a mechanism for dealing with their grief.

For me it has been writing books and developing online emotional support coaching for Carers. I am still learning for myself which means more tools to help others.

What can you give to others that will help you as you go through your own unique grief journey?

<u>CHAPTER 4</u>

Gratitude and Giving

What have I got to be grateful for? I've just lost my loved one!

I write this book during the COVID 19 pandemic when many will find little to be grateful for, especially if you are grieving the passing of a loved one. Or, maybe, you are grieving at not being able to visit them in a Care Home right now.

As I contemplate this and those who may be stuck indoors with a loved one whose diagnosis exhibits challenging behaviour with angry aggressive outbursts; my heart goes out to all those Carers facing what seem insurmountable challenges as a Carer. As well as those on the grieving pathway. With or without the COVID situation the same challenges may be operating in your own experience.

Strange as it may seem, for me it is a blessing that my husband transitioned when he did. I have avoided the emotional trauma of visiting restrictions, especially during the last two weeks of life in the Care Home. This blessing helps me tremendously as I adjust to my new life.

In the world today it seems that humanity has somehow lost sight of the power of gratitude. As the media promotes and focuses on all the negative things in the world, emphasising on fear responses. To find anything to be grateful for can be an uphill struggle.

As I reflect on the last ten years with my man, watching those gradual exacerbated changes with him associated with the cruelty of the Alzheimer's Disease, it could have been easy to lose sight of anything to be grateful for. Watching daily life routine require a different approach, money being sucked out to pay for care, could make one bitter and ungrateful. I am sure my life learnings came into play for which I am grateful and also was along the way. –

- Grateful for a pretty much patient make up looking beyond face value with situations.

- Grateful that in spite of care expenses there was a roof over one's head, food to eat, clothes on one's back plus a car for travelling for appointments and Care Home visits.

- Grateful that there was investment to use for his funding.

These are just a few of my gratitudes. I feel truly blessed that we were provided for.

OK, after his transition, things took quite a different turn, as pension adjustment was "interesting", care funding refused which left a deficit to be settled. Suddenly I am grieving and dealing with some "very interesting" circumstances.

By facing the trials head on and talking to appropriate people and organisations, I was amazed and grateful for the kindness shown to help deal with issues objectively which created solutions.

I have learned that by taking responsibility for unpleasant situations, even when deep sorrow and pain have taken hold, courageously talking to people, brought some amazing solutions that were almost miraculous! Certainly, much has been learned through the last, now eleven years.

- Learning to face situations head on.

- Seeking help and not closing down and hiding away (even if one wanted to).

- Standing strong and objectively negotiating where needed for positive outcomes

- Leaning on my faith in God for peace and guidance.

When going through a very burdensome, emotional roller coaster time, it can seem impossible to be grateful for anything. A powerful habit to create – yes CREATE which takes practice and commitment- is each morning on waking think of one thing you are grateful for.

Maybe it's just being able to somehow get out of bed and put one foot in front of the other.

Maybe it's "today I can grieve well with no judgement"

Maybe it's "my loved one is free of suffering now"

Maybe it's "I can make this a day where it's OK to do only what I want to or can successfully achieve" It may challenge but that is fine. Go for it!

Maybe it's "I am grateful that today I am able to fully express my grief in a way that helps me heal"

Maybe it's "I am grateful that I don't need to feel guilty about being grateful for things as I grieve"

As my second Christmas looms and the usual visit from my older sister is cancelled due to COVID restrictions, I am grateful for us being able to use the power of my Zoom platform and have a "Zoom Christmas lunch!" And "Zoom Teatime".

It can be a real challenge to find things to be grateful for when grief and loss are So high, impacting on the energy to tackle life's essential tasks.

How can the power of giving to others assist with dealing with the overwhelming grief?

I actually made a conscious decision to turn my grief into giving back through books and emotional support coaching for Carers.

Suppose you became a listener for someone else who is grieving – being able to truly empathise because of your own situation. With the power of the internet and mobile phones, there is a great opportunity to send a caring thought out to others. When we give to others, however insignificant we think it may be, it warms the heart and uplifts for a time, relieving the grief pain. Imagine waking up and the first thought could be "in spite of the emotional pain, I got through yesterday so I can get through today".

Think of one thing to be thankful for, whilst not denying you hurt terribly. It may be a day of doing just one or two tasks through the tears. Be grateful for tears that release deep down emotions and use the release tools, expressing your feelings in any way that best suits you and helps with another step forward.

My man was never a gardener - keep the grass cut and that's it! I created borders with shrubs and perennial plants that he enjoyed. As I tend garden now, I talk to him and tell him I am caring for the garden in memory of him. "If you are looking down Brian, I hope you approve of what I am doing". It's like I am creating a beautiful space for visitors to enjoy along with a place to find peace along with reflecting on memories. Autumn brings a smile as I recall the early Alzheimer's days when he looked at the leaves littering the front lawn and cried "Look at all those leaves! I didn't put them there!" I restrained myself from suggesting he reprimand the Canadian Oak trees in our neighbours garden!

Grief is not like a disease you will "recover from". It is a healing of deep emotional wounds that leave scars. Just like a scar can suddenly itch for no reason at all, in the same way grief emotions can rise up. Be there for a reminder of your loved one in that moment. If it is a painful memory, feel and express it, and let it gently fade, thankful that you are allowing your new, adjusted life to be lived.

Never be afraid of reaching out for help and support as there are those who understand and will "be there" for you. Many online support groups are out there – online and phone support has sprung up as a result of the COVID pandemic. Do make sure they are supportive and not a place that will drag you into becoming a grief victim.

Most of all know that with consistent baby steps each day with persistence and gratitude, (for me prayer), you can travel this journey well for You!

CHAPTER 5

If I was to Offer a Few Tips......

Let me start by saying that my tips are primarily from my own experience and people I have met throughout the whole Alzheimer's journey with my husband. I hope they will inspire and help you become a "victorious" griever and not a "victim" griever.

So, let's illustrate the difference between a victim griever and a victorious griever with a couple of examples that certainly illustrate how unique everyone's grief journey is. Plus, in some way can be influenced a great deal by the programming one has received in dealing with day-to-day challenges in life. There is neither condemnation nor congratulation associated with these illustrations – just two very different ways of dealing with the loss of a spouse.

The Victim Journey

A spouse who has been poorly for some time and needed care from their loved one, passes, leaving the Carer feeling alone and grieving the loss of someone very dear to them who played a role of leadership in the marriage with day to day running of the home. Suddenly this has ceased and full responsibility for the day to day upkeep of the home rests solely on the shoulders of the one buried in their grief. Apart from outings for essentials, occasional family visits, they have become almost hermit like. The garden is like a jungle as motivation to take over creating a beautiful space is not there. Their spouse focused on the garden project and there is no way any energy to create in their memory can be mustered up.

The victor Journey

After a long illness in the Dementia arena requiring very sensitive caring input, spouse has suddenly passed away. The pain of grief pops up regularly and seems more intense as time passes. Somehow, they find a way to cope with the pain and tend the garden as a memory project, talking to their loved one as they work, which helps with the healing process.

So, in no special order -

1. Aim at becoming a positive and victorious griever in your own way, own time, accepting others empathy and encouragement along the way.

2. Don't let guilt consume you if you don't follow exactly the "five stages of grief cycle" in an exact order of – denial and isolation, anger, bargaining, depression, acceptance.

3. Make sure that you rest when your body needs it within your own life pattern.

4. Eat regular meals and nourish the body systems. They have been battered through your emotional stress and need support.

5. Get into a daily routine – you may have to indulge in some self- talk regarding getting up each day prepared to walk through your grief with the best self-care possible.

6. Reward yourself when you begin to feel you are progressing through the initial deep hurt and pain.

7. Take a short break on your own when you feel ready to assist with healing the broken heart. Even a walk-in nature or by the sea can be great healing therapy.

8. If it resonates with you, join a support group. While helping you, you may just be the help that someone else needs who is on a similar grief journey.

9. Journal to express and release emotions along with progress steps, no matter how small and seemingly insignificant

10. Keep them "alive" in your heart and thoughts. Moving forward does not mean you have at some point to forget them.

11. It's OK to visit their grave whenever you need if it helps you. Someone once told me that during the first year following her father's

passing, she went to his grave with flowers every week. For her that gave comfort and helped with dealing with her grief.

12. You are unique. Your grief journey is unique to you.

13. "You've done the first year" syndrome does not finalise the adjustment.

14. Be patient with yourself as you grieve.

15. Be honest about how you are feeling. "I'm fine!" Is not always the best response to "How are you doing?". You may choose to say, "I am grieving and adjusting to living well as I move forward".

16. I found a very helpful resource from a Minister and Grief Specialist in the United States named Gary Roe. He has a number of books and grief tools to help those whose hearts have been broken by loss.

OTHER RESOURCES

Sylvia's Website – https://dementia-whisperer.com
For crisis emotional coaching tools, books, free downloads and more.

Alzheimer related books in the trilogy, available on Amazon –

- The Rocky Road of Naughty Neurons
- The Rocky Road of 24/7 Care

From Gary Roe –

Website – www.garyroe.com
For grieving spouse – a book titled Heartbroken, available on Amazon.

ABOUT THE AUTHOR

Sylvia Bryden – Stock is an Accredited Master Coach with a deep trust in the creator of our universe, through Jesus to help us through grieving experiences and blessed to love her wonderful husband against all odds.

Throughout life, her spiritual outlook changed from accepting many ways to find Inner Peace to acknowledging our inner peace that comes from the one true source.

Through her support tools as a dementia whisperer, it is her passion to help others find the way to inner peace and ability to grieve positively and in a way that is unique to them.

It is this approach to life that SO helped Sylvia and can help you with the journey you may be embarking on right now.

www.ingramcontent.com/pod-product-compliance
Lightning Source LLC
Chambersburg PA
CBHW022115050726
47591CB00002B/793